CORE EXERCISES FOR SENIORS

A COMPREHENSIVE GUIDE TO SENIORS FITNESS

NICOLE SMITH

implied endorsement if we use one of these terms.

Table of contents

Conclusion

Introduction

Core exercises are a vital part of any fitness routine, especially for seniors. Strengthening the muscles of the core helps to maintain balance, posture, and mobility, which are important for performing everyday activities. Core exercises can be tailored to any fitness level, from beginner to advanced, making them accessible to seniors of all ages and abilities.

This book is designed to provide you with a comprehensive guide to core exercises that are tailored to the needs of seniors. As you age, it is important to maintain a strong core, which will help you stay balanced and mobile. You will learn how to strengthen your core so you can stay active and fit.

You will also learn exercises that are low-impact and easy to do at home. With this book, you will be able to improve balance, mobility, and strength, and gain a greater sense of well-being and independence. So if you are a senior looking for the best core exercises to stay fit and healthy, this book is for you.

Chapter 1

Understanding core exercises

Core exercises are any type of exercise that engages and strengthens the core muscles of the body. The core muscles are the muscles of the abdomen, lower back, and pelvic floor, and are important for overall stability and balance. Core exercises can help improve posture and balance, as well as reduce the risk of lower back pain and injuries. Core exercises can also help improve performance in sports and other activities by providing a strong foundation for all movement.

The core of your body is the foundation of your strength and stability. As you age, it becomes increasingly important to keep your core strong and stable. Core exercises help to improve balance, posture, and stability.

Core exercises are a great way for seniors to stay active and healthy. Core exercises involve strengthening the muscles of the abdomen, hips, and back, as well as the muscles that support the spine. These muscles help to keep the body balanced and stable, and they can help to prevent falls and injuries.

It is important to understand the different types of core exercises and how they can benefit seniors. Core exercises can be divided into two main categories: static and dynamic.

Static core exercises involve holding a position for several seconds, such as a plank or a bridge. These exercises help to strengthen the core muscles and improve balance.

Dynamic core exercises involve movements such as squats, lunges, and twists. These exercises help to increase the range of motion and improve coordination.

When doing core exercises, it is important to focus on proper form and technique. Begin by performing the exercise with a slow, controlled movement, and gradually increase the intensity as you become more comfortable with the exercise. Make sure to keep your back straight, your core muscles engaged, and your breathing steady.

It is important to remember that core exercises should be done with proper form and technique to prevent injury. It is also important to start slowly and gradually increase the intensity and duration of the exercises as strength and stability improve. It is also important to listen to your body and stop if you experience any pain or discomfort.

It is important to stay consistent with core exercises for seniors to maintain strength and stability. Performing core exercises at least twice per week can help maintain strength and prevent injury. It is also important to consult with your doctor or physical therapist before beginning any exercise program. They can help determine which exercises are most appropriate and safe for you.

Chapter 2

Benefits of core exercises for seniors

1. Improved Posture: Core exercises help strengthen the muscles in the abdomen and lower back, which improves posture and helps prevent back pain.

Improved posture is one of the many benefits of core exercises. Good posture is important for overall health, as it helps to reduce the strain on joints and muscles, as well as improving circulation and breathing. Core exercises help to strengthen the muscles of the torso and spine, which helps to establish better posture.

Core exercises help to improve posture in several ways. First, they help to strengthen the muscles of the torso and spine, which helps to prevent them from becoming weak and weak posture. Strengthening these muscles helps to create a strong foundation for better posture.

Second, core exercises help to improve flexibility and range of motion in the upper body. This improved range of motion will help to improve posture by allowing the body to move more freely and easily.

Third, core exercises help to improve balance and stability in the torso and spine. This improved balance and stability help to create better posture, as the body is better able to support itself.

Finally, core exercises help to improve posture by increasing body awareness. Regular core exercises can help to create a better understanding of how the body is positioned, allowing for better posture when standing, sitting, or walking.

2. Improved Balance and Mobility: Core exercises can help improve balance and coordination, which can help reduce the risk of falls. As people age, their balance can become compromised and they can become more prone to falls and injuries. Core exercises can help to strengthen the muscles in the core area, which can help to improve overall balance and mobility.

The core muscles are responsible for stabilizing the spine, hips, and shoulders, which helps to keep the body in an upright position. By strengthening these muscles, seniors can improve their balance and mobility, and reduce their risk of falls and injuries.

Core exercises can also help to improve coordination and reaction time. By strengthening the muscles in the core area, seniors can increase their range of motion, and make it easier to perform everyday activities, such as bending down to pick something up or reaching for an item on a shelf.

Core exercises can help to improve overall strength and endurance. By strengthening the core muscles, seniors can improve their ability to perform activities of daily living, such as walking, climbing stairs, or carrying groceries. Stronger core muscles can also help to improve overall energy levels, enabling seniors to stay active and engaged in life.

3. Improved Flexibility: Core exercises can help increase flexibility in the spine, hips, and other joints. This can help improve the range of motion and reduce stiffness. Core exercises can help improve balance and stability, which can help seniors stay active and reduce their risk of falls.

Improved flexibility can also help seniors perform everyday tasks more easily and reduce the risk of injury. Core exercises can help seniors increase their range of motion, which can help to reduce joint stiffness and improve posture. Stretching exercises can also help to reduce the risk of muscle strains and other injuries associated with aging. With improved flexibility, seniors can enjoy a more active lifestyle and gain greater independence.

4. Improved Strength and Endurance: Core exercises can help increase strength and endurance, which can help with everyday activities such as carrying groceries, getting up and down from chairs, and walking up stairs. Core exercises can help seniors to maintain and even increase strength and endurance levels during their later years. These exercises target the abdominal, back, and hip muscles, which are vital for balance, posture, and movement.

Strengthening these areas can help to prevent falls and improve stability, which is especially important for seniors who are prone to falling due to age-related changes in muscle strength and balance.

Core exercises can also help to increase energy levels, improve coordination, and reduce the risk of injury. By strengthening the core, seniors can enjoy an increased quality of life and remain active in their later years.

5. Improved Mental Health: Core exercises can help improve mental health by reducing stress, improving focus, and increasing feelings of well-being. Core exercises have been increasingly recognized as an important part of a healthy lifestyle for seniors. Core exercises can help seniors improve their physical health, but researchers have also found that they can also help improve mental well-being.

Core exercises help seniors build strength and balance, which can boost their confidence. This increased confidence can help reduce stress and anxiety levels. Core exercises also help seniors stay active and engaged in activities, which can help them socialize and build relationships with their peers.

In addition, core exercises can help seniors stay focused and can help improve their concentration and memory. These mental benefits can help seniors feel more positive and alert and can improve their overall mental well-being.

Core exercises are an important part of any fitness program, especially for seniors. Core exercises can help to reduce stress and anxiety levels, leading to improved mental well-being. By incorporating core exercises into a senior's fitness routine, they can enjoy the benefits of improved mental well-being and physical health.

6. Improved Quality of Life: Core exercises can help improve quality of life by increasing energy, improving sleep, and reducing fatigue. Core exercises help strengthen the muscles that support the spine, which helps reduce the risk of back pain and improve posture. Stronger core muscles also help seniors move more easily and safely, reducing the risk of falls.

Chapter 3

Creating a routine for core exercises

1. Consult a doctor: As a senior, it is important to create an exercise routine that is tailored to your needs and abilities. It is important to consult with a doctor before beginning any new exercise program. Your doctor can help determine if the exercises you want to perform are safe for your age and health status. They can also provide guidance and advice on how to get the most benefit from your exercise routine. Your doctor can also recommend activities that will help improve your strength, balance, and overall fitness. Consulting with a doctor is a great way to ensure that you are exercising safely and effectively.

2. Make sure the exercises are age and fitness-level-appropriate: Choose exercises that are suited to the individual's physical abilities and limitations. When creating a core exercise routine for seniors, it is important to ensure that the exercises are age and fitness-level appropriate. Exercises that are too difficult or advanced can cause injury or strain, and those that are too easy may not be beneficial.

It is important to consider the physical abilities and limitations of seniors when choosing exercises and to make sure that they can perform the exercises safely and effectively. It is also important to provide modifications whenever necessary and to emphasize proper form and technique. Finally, it is important to provide adequate rest periods and to monitor the intensity of the exercises.

3. Warm-up: When creating a core exercise routine for seniors, it is important to start with a warm-up. Warming up helps to reduce the risk of injury and prepare the body for the exercises ahead. A warm-up should include gentle stretches and/or light aerobic activity to loosen up the muscles and increase the heart rate. It is also important to focus on breathing, as this will help to increase oxygen flow throughout the body. After the warm-up, seniors can then proceed with core exercises like planks, bridges, and side-lying crunches. These exercises will help to strengthen the core muscles, which can help to improve posture and balance.

4. Start with low-impact exercises: Starting with low-impact workouts is a great way for seniors to create a core exercise routine. Low-impact activities such as walking, swimming, and yoga can help strengthen the core muscles without putting too much strain on the body. These exercises can also help improve balance and coordination, which are important for maintaining independence and mobility.

Low-impact exercises are often easier to modify to accommodate any physical limitations or health conditions that may be present. By starting with low-impact exercises, seniors can gradually increase their intensity and complexity as they become more comfortable with the routine.

5. Focus on balance: Creating a routine for core exercises for seniors should focus on balance. Balance exercises can help prevent falls, improve posture, and build strength. Balance exercises can be used to improve range of motion and flexibility. When creating a routine for core exercises for seniors, it is important to remember to start slow and build up with more challenging exercises. Additionally, it is important to ensure that proper form and technique are used.

6. Incorporate strength training: Strength training is an important part of any exercise routine, especially for seniors. Strength training helps maintain muscle mass, bone density, and balance.

Incorporating strength training into a core exercise routine for seniors can help them stay strong, improve their balance and coordination, and reduce the risk of falls.

Strength training exercises should be tailored to the individual's abilities and should include both upper and lower body exercises. It is important to use proper form and technique when performing any strength training exercise to maximize the benefits and avoid injury. It is also important to start at a comfortable level and gradually increase the intensity as strength and endurance improve.

7. Incorporate flexibility exercises: Incorporating flexibility exercises into a core exercise routine for seniors is an important part of maintaining their physical health and well-being. Flexibility exercises help seniors maintain a healthy range of motion in their joints and muscles, which can help reduce the risk of injury from everyday activities. Seniors should incorporate a variety of exercises into their routines to ensure that all muscle groups are challenged and strengthened. Incorporating flexibility exercises into a core exercise routine for seniors can help them to stay healthy and active well into their golden years.

8. Remember to cool down after each exercise session: Remembering to cool down after each section of a core exercise routine is an important part of creating an effective routine for seniors. By cooling down after each section, seniors can prevent any potential injuries that could occur if they were to push themselves too hard.

Cooling down will help seniors stay relaxed and reduce any potential soreness that may occur after the workout. Cooling down also allows seniors to gradually lower their heart rates, which is beneficial for their overall health. Taking a few moments to cool down after each section allows seniors to catch their breath and mentally prepare for the next section of the routine.

9. Have rest days: Rest days are an important part of any exercise routine, especially for seniors. During rest days, seniors can rest their bodies and allow their muscles to recover from the physical exertion of a core exercise routine. Seniors must listen to their bodies and be mindful of when they need to take a break. Rest days help to reduce the risk of injury and soreness, while also allowing seniors to build strength and endurance gradually. Rest days are a great way for seniors to stay healthy and safe while still getting the benefits of a regular exercise routine.

10. Remember to stay hydrated: Staying hydrated is an important part of creating a core exercise routine for seniors. Adequate hydration helps to maintain body temperature, lubricate joints and muscles, transport nutrients, and flush out toxins.

Water is the best choice for hydration and should be consumed throughout the day, not just during exercise. It is recommended that seniors drink at least eight 8-ounce glasses of water per day. During exercise, they should drink water or a sports drink that contains electrolytes. Drinking fluids before, during, and after exercise will help keep seniors hydrated and will help them perform at their best.

Seniors should also be mindful of their sodium intake, as consuming too much sodium can lead to dehydration. Other beverages such as tea, coffee, and sports drinks can be consumed in moderation, but should not replace water as the primary source of hydration.

It is also important for seniors to pay attention to the signs and symptoms of dehydration. These can include feeling dizzy, having a dry or sticky mouth, or feeling unusually tired. If any of these symptoms are noticeable, it is important to immediately stop exercising and seek medical attention.

11. Have fun: Core exercises don't have to be tedious. Try to make it enjoyable by listening to music or doing it with a friend. It is important to keep in mind that seniors are more likely to stick to an exercise routine if it is enjoyable and engaging. Participating in activities that they enjoy and find interesting will help to motivate them to keep up with their routine. Some examples of activities seniors can do to have fun while exercising include dancing, participating in group fitness classes, or playing active games. Incorporating social activities into their routine can help to keep them motivated and engaged. Keeping exercise fun and enjoyable is key for seniors to maintain a healthy lifestyle.

Chapter 4

Beginners core exercises for seniors

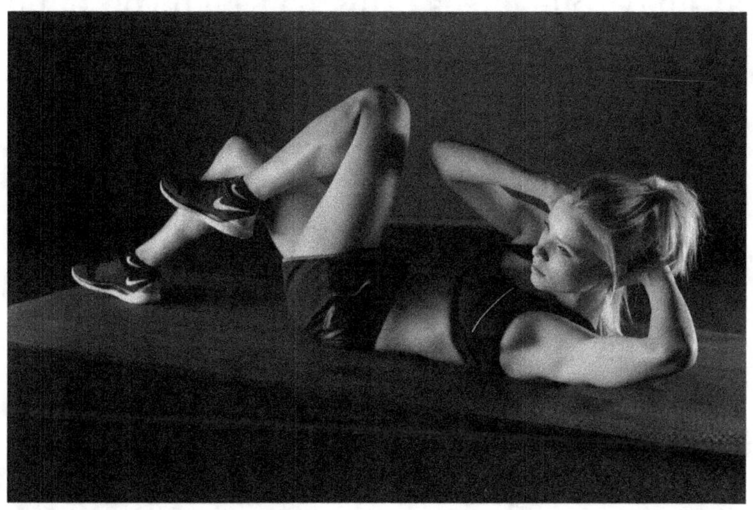

1. Seated Knee Extensions: To do the exercise, you need to start in a kneeling position on the floor with your knees bent and your feet flat on the floor. Then, slowly extend your legs out in front of you, bringing your torso upright and your arms stretched out straight in front of you. Hold this position for a few seconds, before slowly returning to the starting position.

To increase the difficulty of the exercise, you can add ankle weights or a resistance band around your knees. This will help you build strength and improve your balance.

2. Seated Leg Lifts: To perform the exercise, sit on a chair or bench with your legs and feet together, and your back straight. Place your hands on either side of the chair. Lift your legs to the point where your knees and hips form a 90-degree angle. Then, slowly lower your legs back down to the starting position.

Make sure to keep your core engaged and your back straight throughout the exercise.

3. Seated trunk rotations: To perform the exercise, start by sitting on the floor with your legs out in front of you and your feet flat on the floor. Place the hands on the back of the head, then rotate the trunk to the left, going as far as possible without causing pain. Hold for a few seconds before slowly returning to the center and repeating on the right side. Continue alternating sides for 8-10 repetitions.

4. Seated upper body stretches: The key to performing seated upper body stretches is to keep your spine in a neutral position and focus on breathing deeply. Start by sitting upright, engaging your core, and relaxing your shoulders. Then, reach your arms up and out to the sides, keeping your elbows slightly bent. Hold the stretch for 15-30 seconds and repeat 2-3 times.

You can also perform seated upper-body stretches while standing. Reach your arms up and out to the sides and then bring them down to the sides of your body, palms facing forward. Hold the stretch for 15-30 seconds and repeat 2-3 times.

5. Wall sits: To do the wall sit exercise, stand with your back against a wall and your feet shoulder-width apart. Slide your back down the wall until your thighs are parallel to the floor. Keep your feet flat on the floor and your back pressed against the wall. Hold this position for 30-60 seconds, then stand up and repeat.

6. Seated bicep curls: This exercise can be done with a variety of equipment, such as a barbell, dumbbells, resistance bands, or machine weights.

To perform the exercise, you should start by sitting on a bench or chair with your feet planted firmly on the ground. With your arms extended out in front of you, grip the barbell or weight with an underhand grip. With your elbows tucked in close to your sides, slowly curl the weight up towards your shoulder. Once you reach the top of the movement, slowly lower the weight back down to the starting position. Be sure to keep your back straight and your core engaged throughout the entire exercise.

7. Wall squat: It involves standing with your back against a wall and slowly squatting down until your thighs are parallel to the floor. You should hold this position for several seconds before slowly returning to a standing position. This exercise can be modified by changing the amount of time you hold the position, the amount of weight you use, or the type of movement you perform.

8. Seated shoulder shrugs: To do this exercise, sit in a chair with your feet flat on the floor and your back straight. Lift your shoulders towards your ears and hold for a few seconds before releasing. Do 3 sets of 10-15 repetitions.

Remember to keep your feet flat on the ground and your shoulders relaxed. Avoid jerking or bouncing your shoulders during the exercise. Focus on squeezing your shoulder blades together and keeping your chin tucked in.

9. Standing hip bridges: To do this exercise, stand with your feet hip-width apart and your hands on your hips. Bend your knees and lower your hips down into a bridge position. Make sure your back is straight and your core is engaged. Push your hips up and squeeze your glutes at the top of the movement. Hold for a few seconds, then slowly lower back down. Repeat for 10-15 reps.

10. Standing calf raises: The exercise is performed by standing on a raised platform, with your toes pointing forward and your heels hanging off the edge. From this position, you slowly lower your heels towards the floor and then rise back up on the balls of your feet. This exercise can be done with or without weights, depending on your fitness level. It can also be done in a seated position.

11. Seated toe taps: To begin, sit on the edge of the chair or bench with your feet flat on the floor. Keeping your spine straight, slowly lift one foot off the floor and tap your toes to the floor. Make sure to keep your knee bent and your core engaged throughout the exercise. Do 10-15 reps for each leg.

For added intensity, you can add ankle weights to increase the resistance. This exercise can also be done with increased speed for a more challenging workout.

12. Wall push-ups: To perform wall push-ups, stand facing a wall and place your hands on the wall at chest level. Then, bend your elbows and lower your chest towards the wall until your arms are parallel to the floor. Push your body away from the wall until your arms are straight once again. Repeat this motion for 10-15 repetitions.

13. Seated heel raises: To perform the seated heel raise, start by sitting on a firm chair or bench and placing your feet flat on the floor. From here, press through your heels to lift your body off the seat, then slowly lower back down. You can use a lightweight such as a dumbbell to add resistance, or simply use your body weight for a more moderate challenge. Remember to keep your back straight and maintain good posture throughout the movement.

14. Seated arm circles: Keeping your arms straight, slowly moving them in small circles. Start by making 10 circles in one direction, then switch to 10 circles in the other direction. Make sure to move your arms slowly and evenly, and to keep your shoulders relaxed.

You can increase the intensity of the exercise by making larger circles or by using weights. You can also add variety by performing the exercise in a standing position.

15. Kneeling Leg Raises: To perform this exercise, start by kneeling on the floor with your knees slightly wider than hip-width apart. Keep your torso upright and your shoulders relaxed. Engage your core and lift one leg off the floor, using your hip flexors to keep the leg at a 90-degree angle. Hold this position for a few seconds before slowly lowering the leg back to the floor. Repeat on the other side. You can make this exercise more challenging by doing multiple reps or holding a weighted plate. Kneeling leg raises are a great way to strengthen your core and improve your overall balance and coordination.

16. Kneeling Hip Bridges: To do the exercise, start by kneeling on the floor on all fours. Then, raise one leg off the ground and extend it back until the foot is flat on the floor. Keep the other leg bent and the foot flat on the ground. Then, drive the hips up towards the ceiling, squeezing the glutes at the top of the movement. Hold the position for a few seconds and then lower back down. Repeat this exercise on both sides for the desired number of repetitions.

17. Kneeling Side Planks: This exercise can be done as a static hold (holding the position for a set amount of time) or as a dynamic exercise (moving up and down). To perform the exercise, start in a kneeling position with your feet and hips together, then twist your torso to the side and lift your hips off the floor, keeping your body in a straight line. Hold this position for 10-30 seconds, then switch sides. This exercise can be made more challenging by adding weight to your hips or holding the position longer.

18. Lying Glute Bridges: This exercise is performed by lying on your back with your feet flat on the floor and your knees bent. From this position, you slowly lift your hips off the ground, squeezing your glutes as you do so. Hold the bridge position for a few seconds and slowly lower your hips back to the starting position. This exercise can be done with or without weights and can be modified to increase difficulty. It is a great exercise for developing strength and stability in the lower body.

19. Lying Abdominal Crunches: To perform this exercise, first lie on your back with your knees bent and your feet flat on the floor. Place your hands behind your head and gently pull your shoulder blades together. Then, curl your shoulders and upper back off the floor and reach your chest up towards your knees. Hold the position for a few seconds before slowly returning to the starting position.

This exercise can be modified by changing the angle of your legs, the speed of the movement, or the number of repetitions.

20. Lying Leg Lifts: The exercise is performed by lying on your back with your arms outstretched behind you and your legs straight. Then, slowly lift one leg off the ground while keeping the other leg on the ground. Hold this position for a few seconds and then slowly lower the leg back down. Repeat with the other leg and continue alternating sides for the desired amount of repetitions. This exercise can be made more challenging by adding weights or a resistance band.

21. Lying Glute Bridges with Leg Lifts: This exercise requires you to lie on your back, with your knees bent and feet flat on the floor. From this position, you will raise your hips off the floor and hold for a few seconds, then you will lift one leg off the floor and hold for a few seconds. Repeat this for each leg.

22. Lying Hip Raises: To begin, lie on your back with your feet flat on the floor and your knees bent. Place your hands palms down on either side of your body for stability. Engage your core and raise both hips off the floor at the same time. Hold this position for a few seconds before lowering your hips to the floor. Repeat the raise and lower several times.

You can add resistance by holding a lightweight in your hands or by placing a resistance band around your knees. This exercise can also be done with one leg at a time, alternating between each leg.

23. Lying Side-lying Leg Raises: To perform this exercise, lie on one side with your legs and upper body straight. Lift your top leg up and down slowly and steadily, keeping your hips and waist in line with your shoulders. Be sure to keep your core and abdominal muscles engaged throughout the movement. This exercise is a great way to target the abdominal muscles and improve your core stability.

24. Lying Torso Twists: The exercise is performed by lying on your back, with your feet flat on the floor and knees bent. You then twist your torso from side to side, keeping your arms and legs straight throughout the motion. The exercise should be done slowly and with control, and it is important to keep your abdominal muscles contracted and your back flat against the floor.

25. Lying Back Extensions: This exercise is easy to do, requiring only a mat and a comfortable surface. To perform the exercise, start by lying on your stomach with your arms at your sides and your chin slightly tucked in. Slowly lift your upper body off the ground, keeping your arms straight and your neck and shoulders relaxed. Hold this position for a few seconds, then slowly lower your upper body back down. Repeat for 10-15 repetitions.

26. Seated Toe Touches: Seated toe touches are an effective exercise for stretching and strengthening the muscles in the lower body. They target the hamstrings, calves, and glutes, as well as the lower back, and can help improve balance and flexibility. To perform a seated toe touch, begin by sitting on the ground with your legs extended in front of you. Then, slowly reach forward with your fingertips and try to touch your toes. Hold this position for a few seconds, and then slowly bring your hands back towards your body. This exercise can be done as a warm-up or part of a larger stretching routine. Remember to keep your back straight and do not overextend yourself.

27. Seated Arm Raises: This exercise can be done while sitting in a chair or on a bench. To do the exercise, start by sitting up straight and holding your arms out in front of you, palms facing down. Raise your arms and out to the sides until they are parallel to the floor. Hold this position for a few seconds before returning your arms to the starting position. Repeat this exercise 10-15 times for best results.

28. Seated Heel Raises: Seated Heel Raises Exercise is a great way to strengthen your calves and improve your posture. It involves sitting on a chair, with your feet flat on the floor. From this position, you raise your heels off the ground while keeping your toes on the floor. You should hold the raised position for a few seconds before slowly lowering your heels back to the ground. You can repeat this exercise for a few sets of 10 to 20 repetitions.

29. Seated Squats: It is a simple yet effective exercise that can be done at home or in the gym. It targets the quads, glutes, hamstrings, and calves, and can also help improve your balance and core stability. To do the seated squat, sit on a chair or bench with feet flat on the floor, hip-width apart. Push your hips back and bend your knees to lower yourself down until your thighs are parallel to the ground. Hold for a few seconds and then push back up to the starting position. Make sure to keep your chest up and your back straight throughout the exercise. This exercise can be modified by holding weights in your hands or by standing on one leg for an extra challenge.

Chapter 5

Intermediate core exercises for seniors

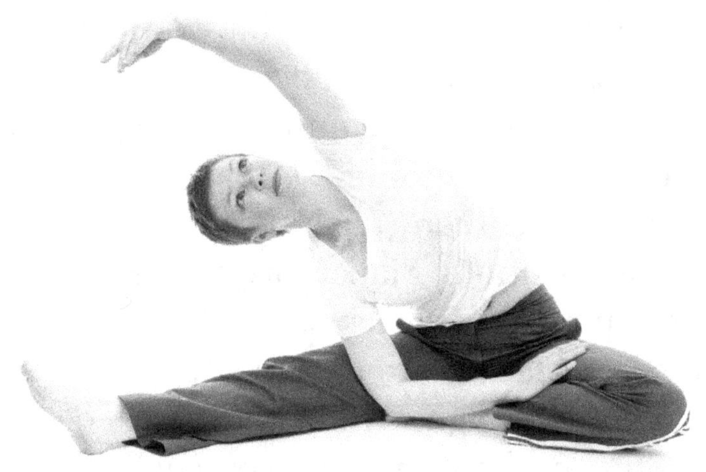

1. Seated Knee Extensions: To do this exercise, start by sitting on the floor with your legs extended in front of you. Place your hands at your side, palms down. Engage your core and slowly slide one of your legs back towards your buttocks, keeping your knee bent. Hold the position for a few seconds, then slowly return to the starting position. Repeat the same movement with the other leg.

Be sure to keep your back straight throughout the exercise and try to keep your hips level. You can increase the difficulty of the exercise by holding a lightweight or medicine ball in your hands.

2. Seated Leg Raises: To perform a seated leg raise, start by sitting with your feet flat on the floor. Lift one leg so your thigh is parallel to the floor and your toes point towards the ceiling. Keep your core muscles engaged and your back straight. Slowly lower the leg to the starting position and repeat with the other leg. Do 10-15 repetitions on each side. For best results, perform the exercise at a steady and controlled pace.

3. Standing Quadriceps Stretch: The standing quadriceps stretch is an effective exercise to improve flexibility in the muscles of the thigh. It is a simple, yet effective way to reduce tightness and improve the range of motion in the quad muscles.

To begin, stand up straight and hold onto a stationary object for balance. Bend your left leg and grab your left ankle with your left hand. Pull your ankle up and back until you feel a stretch in the front of your thigh. Hold this position for 15-30 seconds. Switch sides and repeat.

This exercise should be done regularly to maintain flexibility and range of motion in the thighs.

4. Standing Calf Stretch: Standing Calf Stretch Exercise is a great way to help improve flexibility and strength in the calf muscles. This exercise is easy to do and can be done almost anywhere. To start the exercise, stand facing a wall or other stable surface. Place one foot slightly behind the other and press your toes against the wall. Bend the front knee slightly and press your heel into the floor. Hold for 30 seconds and then switch legs. Make sure to keep your back straight and your core engaged throughout the stretch.

5. Seated Toe Touches: It helps to strengthen your core and lower body muscles, while also stretching your hamstrings and calves. To do the exercise, start by sitting on the floor with your legs straight out in front of you. Reach your arms up and over your head, and then slowly lean forward, trying to reach your toes with your fingertips. Hold the stretch for a few seconds and then slowly return to your starting position. Repeat the exercise several times to complete one set.

6. Standing Hamstring Stretch: To perform this exercise, stand with your feet shoulder-width apart. Hold onto a wall, chair, or counter for support. Bend your right knee and raise your right foot off the floor, keeping your knee bent. Gently push your hips forward until you feel a stretch in the back of your right leg. Hold this position for 10-15 seconds, then switch sides.

This exercise can be performed daily to help improve hamstring flexibility. Be sure to use slow and gentle motions, and listen to your body to avoid any discomfort or pain.

7. Seated Heel Lift: To perform this exercise, sit on a chair with feet firmly planted on the floor. Lift your heels as far as you can, then slowly lower them back to the floor. Make sure to keep your toes in contact with the ground. Do 10-15 repetitions of this exercise, taking a few seconds to rest between each one.

This exercise is great for improving balance, coordination, and posture, as well as strengthening and toning your lower body. It's also a great way to relieve tension in the lower body after a long day of standing or walking.

8. Seated Trunk Rotation: The exercise involves sitting in a chair and rotating the torso from side to side. This can be done with a weight or without.

9. Standing Back Bend: To perform this exercise, start by standing with your feet shoulder-width apart. Then, take a deep breath in, and on the exhale, begin to reach your arms up and back, arching your back as you reach. Be sure to keep your neck in line with your spine, and your core engaged. Hold the position for up to a minute, and then return to standing.

This exercise can be quite difficult and may cause some discomfort. If so, be sure to stop the exercise and modify it to accommodate your current level of flexibility and strength.

10. Seated Spinal Twist: To do the seated spinal twist, first sit on the floor with your legs straight out in front of you and your spine in a neutral position. Place your left hand behind you on the floor and reach your right arm across your body to the outside of your left knee. Gently twist your torso to the left, feeling the stretch in your back and abdominals. Hold the twist for a few breaths, then release and repeat on the other side.

Make sure to keep your spine neutral and your chest open, and don't force the twist beyond what is comfortable.

11. Standing Wall Squats: To do this exercise, stand with your back against a wall and bend your knees until your thighs are parallel to the floor. Hold this position for 10 to 30 seconds, then stand back up. Make sure to keep your back flat against the wall and your knees in line with your toes.

Repeat this exercise for 1-3 sets of 8-12 repetitions. For a more challenging version, hold a medicine ball or a dumbbell in front of your chest while doing the exercise.

12. Seated Hip Abduction: To perform seated hip abduction exercises, sit on a chair or bench with your feet flat on the floor. Place a band around the thighs just above the knees and slowly lift one leg up and away from the body. Hold for a few seconds, then slowly lower the leg back down to the starting position. Repeat on the other side. Make sure to keep your back straight and your feet flat on the floor throughout the exercise.

13. Standing Side Bends: To do the exercise, stand with your feet shoulder-width apart and your hands on your hips. Slowly bend your body to one side, then return to the starting position. Make sure to keep your back straight and your hips level throughout the exercise. Repeat the move on the other side.

Perform 10-20 repetitions of the standing side bends exercise on each side. If you feel comfortable doing more, you can increase the repetitions as you become stronger.

14. Seated Pelvic Tilts: To do the exercise, start by sitting up straight in a chair with your feet flat on the floor. Place your hands on your hips and then tilt your pelvis forward, pushing your lower back into the chair. Hold the tilt for a few seconds and then return to the starting position. Repeat the exercise 10-15 times.

15. Standing Glute Squeeze: It involves standing with feet hip-width apart and squeezing the glutes together while maintaining a neutral spine. The exercise can be done with or without weights and is a great way to strengthen the glutes, improve posture, and build balance and stability.

16. Seated Hip Flexor Stretch: To begin, sit on the edge of a chair or bench with your feet flat on the ground and your knees bent. Slowly lift one knee towards your chest, then lower it back down. Repeat with the other knee and continue for 10-12 reps. Make sure to keep your core engaged and your back straight throughout the exercise. This exercise can be made more challenging by adding weights or resistance bands for additional resistance.

17. Standing Shoulder Press: To perform the standing shoulder press, begin by standing with your feet shoulder-width apart and your core engaged. Hold a barbell in front of your chest with your palms facing away from you. Slowly press the barbell up and overhead until your arms are extended and the barbell is directly above your head. Pause at the top, then slowly lower the barbell back to the starting position.

The standing shoulder press can be performed with either a barbell or dumbbell and is a great exercise for building shoulder strength and stability.

18. Seated Shoulder Retraction: To perform the seated shoulder retraction exercise, sit up tall in the chair with your feet flat on the floor. Place your hands on your upper back, slightly above the shoulder blades. Gently squeeze your shoulder blades together and hold for 5 seconds. Relax and repeat this motion 10 times.

19. Standing Arm Circles: To do this exercise, stand with your feet hip-width apart and arms extended out to the side at shoulder height. Begin by slowly rotating your arms in circles, making sure to keep your arms straight and your chest up. Continue for 30 to 60 seconds, then switch directions.

This exercise is great for both beginners and advanced exercisers. It can be done with or without weights, and the speed of the circles can be increased or decreased as you progress.

20. Seated Arm Raises: This exercise involves sitting in a chair with your feet flat on the floor and your hands by your sides. You then lift your arms out to the sides as high as you can, keeping your elbows slightly bent. You should feel the tension in your shoulder muscles as you do this. Hold this position for a few seconds before slowly lowering your arms back down. Repeat this exercise for a total of 10-15 repetitions. This is a great exercise to incorporate into your workout routine.

21. Standing Abdominal Crunches: It is a simple exercise that can be done anywhere with minimal equipment. To do a standing abdominal crunch, stand with your feet shoulder-width apart and place your hands behind your head. Keeping your back straight, bend at the waist and crunch your upper body until your shoulder blades are nearly touching. Hold this position for a few seconds before returning to the starting position. You can make the exercise more challenging by adding weights.

22. Seated Leg Lifts: To perform the exercise, sit in a chair with your feet flat on the floor. Place your hand's palms down on either side of your hips for support. Lift one leg straight out in front of you, keeping your knee slightly bent. Hold for a few seconds, then lower your leg back to the starting position. Repeat with your other leg.

Do 8 to 12 repetitions of this exercise on each leg. For best results, perform 3 sets of the exercise.

23. Standing Side Leg Raises: The basic movement of the exercise is to raise one leg off the ground, keeping the other leg bent, and then lower the leg back to the ground in a controlled manner. You can use a resistance band to add resistance to the exercise and make it more challenging. As you do this exercise, focus on keeping your core tight and your back straight.

24. Seated Heel Raises: To do this exercise, sit on the edge of a chair with your feet flat on the floor. Slowly raise your heels off the ground and hold for a few seconds before lowering them back down. Repeat this exercise 10-15 times, depending on your fitness level.

25. Seated Calf Raises: To perform this exercise, you start seated on a bench or chair with your feet flat on the floor. Keeping your knees bent, press through your toes to raise your heels off the floor, then slowly lower them back down. You can increase the difficulty of the exercise by adding some weight, such as by holding a dumbbell or kettlebell in each hand.

26. Standing Toe Raises: To do a standing toe raise, stand with your feet shoulder-width apart and your toes pointing straight ahead. Slowly raise one foot off the ground and hold it for a few seconds. Then lower it back to the ground and repeat with the other foot.

Be sure to keep your back straight and your toes pointed straight ahead throughout the exercise. You can also add a light dumbbell or resistance band to add extra intensity.

27. Seated Ankle Rotations: exercise is performed while seated in a chair with feet firmly planted on the floor. The torso is then rotated from side to side in a controlled manner. It is important to keep the trunk and neck in proper alignment during the exercise, as well as to move through a full range of motion. Additionally, the use of light weights or resistance bands can be added to increase the intensity of the exercise. Seated Angle Rotation is a great way to increase spinal mobility, improve core strength, and reduce the risk of back pain and injury.

28. Standing Core Rotations: To do this exercise, stand with your feet shoulder-width apart and your arms extended out to the side. Rotate your torso and arms to one side, then back to the starting position, and repeat on the other side. Make sure you keep your core tight throughout the entire exercise and keep your movements slow and controlled. If you're looking for an additional challenge, you can add a medicine ball, weight plate, or resistance band to increase the difficulty.

29. Seated Oblique Twist: To perform the exercise, sit on the floor with your legs crossed and your feet flat on the ground. Place the hands behind the head and twist the torso to one side, then back to the center, and then to the other side. Make sure to keep the back straight throughout the movement. Repeat the movement for 10-15 repetitions on each side.

This exercise can be made more challenging by adding a weight or a medicine ball to the exercise, or by increasing the number of repetitions. This exercise can also be done standing, using a cable machine or a resistance band.

Overall, the seated oblique twist is a great exercise for strengthening the core and toning the abdominals. It is also a great way to improve posture and balance.

30. Standing Back Extension: Standing back extension exercise is a great way to strengthen your back muscles, particularly the lower back. It is an effective way to improve your posture and reduce back pain.

To do the exercise, stand with your feet shoulder-width apart and your arms by your sides. Bend your knees slightly and hinge forward at your hips while keeping your chest up and your back flat. Keep your arms straight and your head in line with your spine. Push your hips back and slowly lift your arms behind you as high as you can. Hold at the top for a moment before slowly returning to the starting position.

Make sure to keep your core engaged throughout the exercise, and focus on using your back muscles rather than your arms. Start with 10-15 repetitions and increase the number as you become more comfortable with the exercise.

31. Seated Bent-Knee Push-Ups: To do a seated bent knee push-up, sit on the floor with your legs bent and feet flat on the ground. Place your hands on the floor slightly wider than shoulder-width apart and keep your back straight. Slowly lower your chest towards the floor while keeping your elbows close to your body. As you lower your chest, keep your core tight and your glutes engaged. Push away from the floor until your arms are straight, then repeat.

32. Standing Abdominal Twists: To do this exercise, stand with your feet shoulder-width apart and your arms extended out to your sides. Slowly twist your torso from side to side, reaching as far as you can with your arms. Keep your head and chest upright and your back straight. You can add resistance by holding a weight or medicine ball in your hands.

Make sure to keep your breathing steady throughout the exercise and to focus on your form. To maximize the benefit of this exercise, repeat the twist 10-15 times on each twist

33. Seated Balance Push-Ups: This exercise is performed while seated on the floor, with your hands in a push-up position. You then press your body up and down while keeping your balance, as if you were doing a regular push-up. This exercise is great for building strength and improving your balance and stability. It can also be used as a warm-up or cool-down for other exercises. To make this exercise more challenging, you can add a medicine ball or other weight to increase the difficulty. Seated balance push-ups are a great way to improve your overall fitness.

34. Standing Single-Leg Balance: Standing Single Leg Balance Exercise is an effective exercise to improve balance and stability. This exercise requires you to stand on one leg with the other leg raised off the ground and your arms extended straight out from your sides. You should maintain this position for as long as you can while focusing on maintaining your balance.

35. Seated Heel-To-Butt Squeezes: To perform the exercise, sit on the floor with your knees bent and feet flat on the floor.

Place both hands behind the head and interlock the fingers. Inhale and, as you exhale, squeeze the glutes and hamstrings while bringing the heels in towards the buttocks. Hold the contraction for a few seconds, then slowly return to the starting position. Repeat for the desired number of reps.

36. Standing Core Squeezes: To do this exercise, stand with your feet hip-width apart and your arms by your sides. Squeeze your abdominal muscles and glutes, drawing your navel in towards your spine. Hold this position for a few seconds, then relax. Repeat this process several times.

37. Seated Core Tap: To do a seated core tap, begin by sitting on the floor with your legs bent and your feet flat on the ground. Place your hands behind your head and your elbows pointing outwards. Lift your chest slightly, engaging your core muscles, and slowly move your left elbow towards your right knee. Return to the starting position and repeat with your right elbow towards your left knee.

Repeat this exercise for 10-15 repetitions, taking care to keep your back straight and your elbows pointed outwards. Make sure to keep your core engaged throughout the movement. This exercise can be done as part of a larger core workout or as a stand-alone exercise. Try to perform 2-3 sets of the exercise for maximum benefit.

38. Seated Shoulder Extensions: To perform a seated shoulder extension exercise, begin by sitting in a chair with your feet flat on the floor. Place your hands on the back of the chair and slowly bend your elbows to lower your chest towards the floor. Then, press your hands down and extend your arms, pushing your chest up and away from the chair. Keep your elbows close to your body throughout the exercise.

Repeat for 10-15 repetitions and perform 2-3 sets. You can also add resistance to the exercise by holding a lightweight or resistance band in your hands. As you become more comfortable with the movement, increase the repetitions and resistance.

39. Standing Knee Hugs: To perform this exercise, stand with your feet shoulder-width apart and your arms at your sides. Then, lift your right knee towards your chest, while keeping your left leg straight. Wrap your arms around your right knee and give it a gentle hug. Hold this position for a few seconds, then release and repeat on the other side. This exercise can be done as a single rep or repeated multiple times for a more intense workout.

40. Seated Dynamic Arm Circles: To perform this exercise, sit upright on a bench or chair with your feet flat on the floor. Place your hands on your hips and slowly make small circles with your shoulders, alternating directions. Make sure you keep your arms straight and your head and neck in a neutral position. Continue for 30-60 seconds and repeat as needed.

41. Standing Core Plank: To do the Standing Core Plank Exercise, stand with feet slightly wider than hip-width apart and place your hands on your hips. Engage your abdominal muscles and slowly lower your body into a low plank position by bending your knees and pushing your hips back. Make sure your body is in a straight line from your head to your ankles. Hold for 30 to 60 seconds and then slowly return to the starting position.

42. Seated Core Rotations: To perform the Seated Core Rotation exercise, begin by sitting up straight in a chair. Place your feet flat on the floor and your hands on the sides of the chair. Inhale and slowly rotate your torso to one side while keeping your hips, shoulders, and head facing forward. Hold this position for a few seconds before slowly returning to the starting position.

Repeat this exercise 10-15 times on each side. You can also increase the intensity by holding a medicine ball or dumbbell in your hands as you rotate. This will further engage the core muscles and help to improve your overall strength and stability.

43. Standing Marching: To perform the exercise, stand with your feet shoulder-width apart and your hands on your hips. Lift one leg and bend it up towards your chest. As you do, bring the opposite arm up in the air. Alternate legs and arms as you march in place. Focus on keeping your back straight and your core engaged.

The standing marching exercise can be done for a few minutes a day, or it can be incorporated into a longer workout. As your strength and endurance improve, you can increase the speed of the march or add some jumps or skips to the routine.

44. Seated Wall Sits: This exercise involves sitting against a wall with your legs bent at a 90-degree angle and your back flat against the wall. You will then lower yourself down as far as you can while keeping your back and head against the wall. Hold this position for as long as you can and then return to the starting position. This exercise works to build strength in your legs, glutes, core, and upper body. It can also help to improve balance and posture.

45. Standing Wall Push-Ups: To do a standing wall push-up, stand facing a wall with your feet about shoulder-width apart. Place your hands on the wall at about shoulder height and press your body away from the wall. Bend your elbows and lower your chest towards the wall until your nose touches the wall. Push back up to the starting position, keeping your body straight.

You should do at least 10 reps of this exercise to get the most out of it. As you get stronger, you can increase the reps or add additional sets. The standing wall push-up is a great way to build upper body strength and can be done almost anywhere.

46. Seated Arm and Leg Raises: Seated arm and leg raises are a great exercise for improving core strength and balance. They involve sitting on a chair or bench with your feet flat on the ground and your hands on the armrests. From this position, you lift your arms straight up and then your legs straight out in front of you. You can also alternate between the two, doing one move with your arms and then one move with your legs.

47. Standing Balance Reach: This exercise can be performed while standing on one leg, or with both legs together. To perform this exercise, start by standing with your feet hip-width apart and your arms at your sides. Reach your right arm up and across your body towards your left side, while lifting your left leg off the ground. Hold this position for a few seconds, then reach your left arm up and across your body towards your right side, while lifting your right leg off the ground. Hold this position for a few seconds, then return to your starting position. Repeat this exercise for 10-15 repetitions on each side.

48. Seated Glute Bridge: This exercise is performed by sitting on the floor with your knees bent and feet flat on the ground. Then, you drive your hips up off the floor while squeezing your glutes, hold the peak contraction for a few seconds, and then slowly lower back down. This exercise can be done with a resistance band or without and can be progressed by adding weight to

the exercise by holding a weighted plate on
your hips.

Chapter 6

Advanced core exercises for seniors

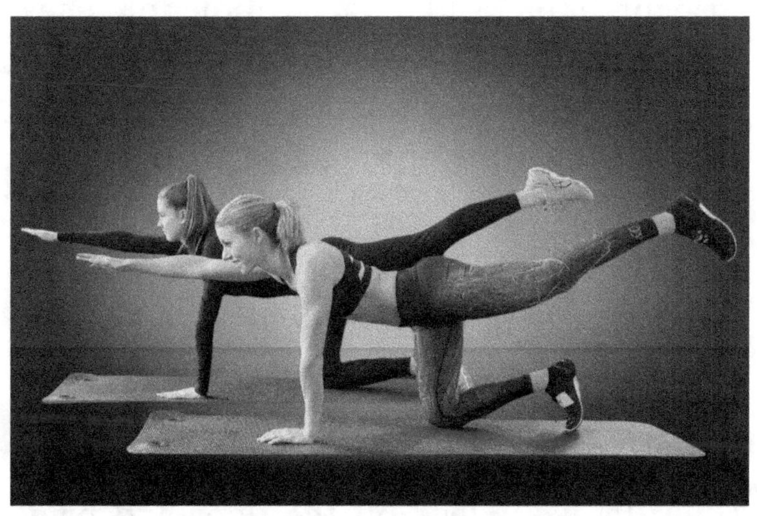

1. Bird Dog: To do the bird dog exercise, start on all fours with your hands directly under your shoulders and your knees directly under your hips. Lift your opposite arm and leg so that your body forms a straight line. Hold this position for a few seconds and then slowly lower your arm and leg back to the starting position. Repeat the exercise with the opposite arm and leg.

2. Seated Knee Lifts: The seated knee lift exercise can be done with or without weights depending on your fitness level. To do the exercise, start by sitting on the floor and leaning back slightly on your hands. Then, lift your legs off the floor and bring your knees up towards your chest. Hold the position for a few seconds and then slowly lower your legs back down to the floor. Repeat the exercise 8-15 times for 1-3 sets. This exercise can help improve core strength and stability, as well as help you get stronger.

3. Seated Kickbacks: The exercise is performed while seated on a bench or stability ball with your back flat and core engaged. You then lift your leg and kick it back behind you in a controlled manner. This exercise should be done slowly and with control to ensure proper form and maximize the benefits. Make sure to keep your core engaged and back flat throughout the entire Kickback

4. Chair Squats: To perform chair squats, begin by standing with your feet hip-width apart and your arms at your sides. Next, slowly lower your body by bending at the hips and knees and sitting back in the chair. Make sure to keep your chest up and your back straight. Once you are in the seated position, pause for a few seconds before pushing back up to the starting position. You can increase the intensity of the exercise by holding weights or by standing on an exercise step.

5. Wall Sits: To perform a wall sit, start by standing with your back against a wall. Slowly slide your back down the wall until your thighs are parallel to the ground and your knees are bent at a 90-degree angle. Hold this position for as long as you can, aiming for at least 30-45 seconds. As your muscles fatigue, be sure to maintain good posture and keep your back flat against the wall. Wall sits are a great way to build strength and endurance in your lower body and can be performed anywhere and at any time.

6. Seated Chair Rotations: To do the exercise, start by sitting in a chair with your feet flat on the floor and your arms on the armrests. Then, slowly rotate your upper body to the left and right, keeping your hips and legs facing forward. Make sure to keep your spine in a neutral position and keep your head aligned with your shoulders. Repeat this exercise for 10-15 repetitions before switching sides. Seated chair rotation can be done as part of a regular stretching routine or as a way to warm up before a workout.

7. Seated Reverse Flys: To do this exercise, sit on a bench with your feet flat on the floor and your knees bent. Hold a pair of dumbbells or resistance bands in front of your thighs with your palms facing toward your inner thighs. Slowly raise the weights out to the sides of your body until your arms are parallel to the floor. Keep your chest up and back straight as you move your arms. Pause for a second in this position before slowly returning to the starting position. Repeat for the desired number of repetitions.

8. Standing Leg Extensions: To do this exercise, stand with your feet hip-width apart and hold a weight in each hand. Keeping your back straight and your knees slightly bent, lift your right leg out to the side and up, then lower it back down.

Repeat with the left leg. Aim for 15 reps on each side.

This exercise can be done with or without weights, depending on your fitness level. Start with a lighter weight and increase it as you get stronger. Make sure to keep your body in a straight line and your core engaged throughout the exercise.

9. Standing Arm Raises: To perform Standing Arm Raises, stand with your feet shoulder-width apart and your arms at your sides. Raise your arms straight out to the sides until they are parallel to the floor. Make sure to keep your elbows slightly bent. Hold for a count of two and then release.

Repeat this exercise for 10-15 repetitions. Increase the number of repetitions as your strength and flexibility improve.

10. Standing Toe Touches: Standing toe touches is an exercise that helps to strengthen the core, improve balance, and increase flexibility. It is a great way to warm up before a workout or to cool down after one. To perform a standing toe touch, stand with your feet shoulder-width apart and your arms at your sides. Raise your arms above your head and reach toward your toes. Hold this position for a few seconds and then return your arms to your sides. Repeat the exercise 10-15 times.

11. Side Steps with Band: To do this exercise, start by standing on the band with your feet shoulder-width apart and the band around your ankles. Then, take a step to the side with your right foot and then bring your left foot to the same position. Alternate between each foot, stepping to the right and then to the left. Make sure to keep your feet slightly wider than shoulder-width apart to ensure that you're getting the full range of motion.

12. Tricep Dips: This exercise can be done using a bench or chair, and can be done with or without weights. To do a tricep dip, start by sitting on the edge of the bench or chair, with your hands placed shoulder-width apart on the edge. Lift your body off the bench, keeping your arms straight and your body close to the bench. Slowly lower your body down until your elbows are bent at a 90-degree angle, and then press back up. Repeat for the desired number of repetitions. It is important to keep your back straight and your shoulders down throughout the exercise.

13. Bent-Over Rows: To perform a bent-over row, begin by standing with your feet hip-width apart and your knees slightly bent. Hinge forward from your hips, keeping your back flat and your core engaged. Grip a barbell (or dumbbell) with an overhand grip, palms facing down. Squeeze your shoulder blades together and pull the barbell (or dumbbells) up towards your chest. Make sure your elbows stay close to your body throughout the movement. Lower the barbell (or dumbbells) back down to the starting position and repeat.

14. Seated Row with Band: To perform this exercise, sit upright on the floor with your legs extended in front of you, and your feet against the anchor point of the band or cable machine. Grab the band or cable handle with both hands and pull it towards your chest, squeezing your shoulder blades together. Slowly return to the starting position and repeat for the desired number of repetitions. This exercise can be made more challenging by adding additional resistance or by performing the exercise on an incline.

15. Plank with Alternating Leg Lifts: The exercise involves holding a basic plank position while alternating lifting one leg at a time. To do this exercise correctly, begin by getting into a plank position on the floor.

Make sure your back is straight and your body is in a straight line from your shoulders to your heels. Then, lift one leg off the ground and hold it for a few seconds. Lower the leg and then switch to the other side. Keep alternating for 30 seconds to 1 minute depending on your fitness level.

16. Lateral Band Walks: The exercise involves placing a resistance band around your ankles while in a plank position. You then take lateral steps with each leg while keeping your core tight and your hips level.

17. Single-Leg Deadlifts: To perform the single-leg deadlift, stand on one leg with the opposite leg slightly bent and raised off the ground behind you. Keeping your back straight and your core tight, slowly hinge at the hip as you lower your upper body toward the floor. As you go down, keep your raised leg straight, and use your hands to help you balance if necessary. When you feel a stretch in your working leg, pause and then drive through your heel to return to the starting position.

18. Squat Jumps: Squat Jumps are a great full-body workout that targets both your lower body and core muscles. They involve squatting down and then jumping up as high as you can. When doing squat jumps, make sure to keep your back straight and your core engaged. Also, land with your feet apart and slightly wider than hip-width apart. Keep your arms and hands at your sides, and try to keep your feet on the ground for as long as possible.

19. Glute Bridges: To do a glute bridge, start by lying on your back with your knees bent and feet flat on the floor. Then, lift your hips off the floor, squeezing your glutes at the top, before slowly returning to the starting position. Be sure to keep your core engaged throughout the exercise, and focus on engaging your glutes as you lift and lower your hips.

20. Step-Ups: To begin, stand in front of a stair or step and place one foot on the step. Push off your front foot and step up onto the step, bringing the other foot up as well. Lower back down and repeat with the opposite foot. Keep your core engaged, chest up, and back straight throughout the exercise. As you become more comfortable, you can increase the height of the step or add weights.

21. Lunges: To perform lunges, stand with your feet hip-width apart, then take a large step forward with your right foot and lower your body until both knees are bent at a 90-degree angle. Keep your torso upright and your weight on your heel as you push up to return to the starting position. Repeat with the left leg.

22. Calf Raises: The exercise works by raising and lowering your body weight on the balls of your feet. This movement can be done with just body weight or with additional weight such as dumbbells or a barbell. To perform a calf raise, stand with your feet hip-width apart and your toes and balls of your feet on the ground. Keeping your legs straight, slowly raise your heels as high as you can. Then, lower your heels back to the starting position. Make sure to keep your legs straight and core engaged throughout the movement.

23. Standing Heel Raises: In the standing heel raises exercise, start by standing with your feet flat on the ground. Bend your knees slightly and raise your heels off the ground. Hold the position for a few seconds and then lower your heels back down to the ground. Repeat the exercise for the desired number of repetitions.

24. Toe Raises: To do the exercise, stand on your toes with your feet together and your arms out. Make sure to keep your back straight and your abs tight. Hold this position for 30 seconds, then relax and repeat. As you become more comfortable with the exercise, try increasing the amount of time you can hold the position. Remember to keep your breathing steady and stay focused on your form.

25. Plank with Arm Raises: To do the plank with arm raises, start in a plank position with your legs straight, arms straight, and hands directly under your shoulders. Engage your core and glutes to keep your body in a straight line. From this position, slowly lift your right arm off the ground and raise it in front of you until your arm is parallel to the ground. Hold for a few seconds, then slowly lower it back to the starting position. Repeat with the left arm. Do 10-15 repetitions for 2-3 sets.

26. Wall Walks: To perform a wall walk, stand with your back against a wall, feet facing forward, and shoulder width apart. Slowly walk your feet up the wall, taking your hands off the wall if possible. Once you are in a handstand position against the wall, hold for a few seconds and then walk your feet back down the wall. Repeat this exercise for 3-5 sets of 10-15 repetitions. For more challenges, you can add additional

27. Mountain Climbers: Mountain Climbers is a full-body, cardiovascular exercise that works your core and leg muscles. It is a great exercise to help you build strength, increase endurance, and burn fat. This exercise can be done by almost anyone and can be adapted to any fitness level.

To do this exercise, start in a plank position with your hands and feet on the ground. Then, drive one knee up towards your chest while keeping the other leg straight. Alternate legs and continue this motion for 30-60 seconds. Mountain Climbers can be an intense workout, so remember to take breaks as needed.

28. Modified push-ups: Modified Push-Ups are a great way to build strength and endurance without putting too much strain on your joints and muscles. They are a great option for those who are new to exercise or who are trying to increase their strength without putting too much strain on their bodies. Modified Push-Ups are done by starting in a kneeling position, with your hands on the floor in front of you. Keeping your back straight and core engaged, slowly lower your chest towards the floor. Pause at the bottom before pushing back up to the starting position. This exercise can be made easier or harder by changing the angle of your body and can be adapted to any skill level.

29. Burpees: They involve squatting down, jumping up, and then coming back down into a squatting position.

30. Balance reach: They involve standing on one leg and reaching with the opposite hand to touch a specified object, such as a wall or chair.

31. plank holds: The exercise involves maintaining a plank position for an extended time, usually 30 seconds or more. This can be done by getting into a plank position with your arms and legs straight out, your feet together, and your head and neck in a neutral position. You should focus on keeping your core and glutes tight during the exercise and make sure that your hips and shoulders remain level.

32. Reverse lunges: To perform a Reverse Lunge, stand tall with your feet hip-width apart and your hands on your hips. Step back with your left leg, keeping your toes pointed forward and your left knee bent at a 90-degree angle. Lower your body towards the ground until your right thigh is parallel to the ground, keeping your core engaged and your chest up. Push off your left leg to return to the starting position. Repeat the same movement on the other side.

33. Pilates: Pilates is an excellent core workout for seniors because it provides a low-impact, full-body strengthening, and toning workout. It promotes mobility, flexibility, balance, and coordination, which can be especially beneficial for older adults. It can also increase strength, improve posture, and reduce the risk of falls and injuries.

The core muscles are the foundation of the body and play a crucial role in everyday activities such as walking, sitting upright, and reaching and lifting objects. Pilates is a great way to target those muscles and help seniors maintain their independence.

Pilates exercises focus on controlled and precise movements that isolate and strengthen the core muscles. This helps to improve posture, stabilize the spine, and prevent injuries. It also increases balance and coordination, which can be especially beneficial for seniors as they age.

The slow and gentle movements of Pilates can be easily adapted to any fitness level, making it a great choice for seniors. It can be done in the privacy of their own homes, or a group setting such as a Pilates class.

Pilates can provide a huge range of physical and mental benefits for seniors. It can help to improve balance, build strength, reduce the risk of falls and injuries, and improve mood and quality of life.

Overall, Pilates is an excellent core workout for seniors and can help them stay active and independent as they age. It is low-impact, can be tailored to any fitness level, and can provide a range of physical and mental benefits.

34. Yoga: Yoga is an excellent core exercise for seniors for many reasons. Not only does yoga strengthen and tone the core muscles, but it also helps to improve balance and flexibility, both of which can be beneficial for seniors as they age. Additionally, yoga can help to reduce stress and improve overall mental health, which are important aspects of aging gracefully. Finally, yoga is a low-impact exercise, meaning it is gentle on the joints and can be done without fear of injury. For these reasons, yoga is an ideal core exercise for seniors.

Chapter 7

Safety tips for core exercises

As we age, our bodies become more fragile and more prone to injury. This means that it's more important than ever for seniors to take extra precautions when it comes to exercise and fitness. Core exercises, in particular, can be especially beneficial for seniors, helping to improve strength, balance, and stability. However, seniors should take special care when performing core exercises to ensure they are done safely and in the proper form.

Here are some safety tips for seniors to keep in mind when performing core exercises:

1. Start slow: Don't rush into any exercise. Start with a few basic exercises and gradually increase the intensity as your body becomes more accustomed to them. As a senior, it is important to begin slowly and gradually increase the intensity of your workouts. Starting too quickly can cause injury or strain to your muscles and joints. Start with low-impact activities such as walking, swimming, or biking. Build up your endurance and strength gradually over time. Make sure to always warm up your muscles and joints before exercising.

2. Warm-up: Before performing any core exercises, it's important to warm up your body by doing some light stretching and aerobic exercise. Warming up helps to loosen up your muscles and increases the circulation of blood in your body. It is recommended to start with a light warm-up like walking or jogging for five to ten minutes before starting any more strenuous exercise. This will help to prepare your body for the workout and reduce the risk of injuries.

3. Use the correct amount of weight: If you are just starting, it's important to use the correct amount of weight for your level of fitness. Start with lighter weights and gradually increase the weight as your core muscles become stronger.

4. Don't overdo it: It's important to challenge yourself, but don't push too hard. Listen to your body and don't attempt exercises that may be too difficult for you.

5. Take breaks: Give yourself rest days between workouts. This will allow your body to recover and reduce the risk of injury. If something doesn't feel right or you're experiencing pain, stop the exercise.

6. Use a mat or cushion: It's important to make sure you're comfortable when performing core exercises. A mat or cushion can help make your workouts more comfortable and reduce the risk of straining your body.

By following these safety tips, seniors can enjoy the many benefits of core exercises while reducing the risk of injury. Core exercises can help to improve balance, stability, and overall strength, but it's important to take the proper precautions to ensure that you are doing them safely.

Conclusion

In conclusion, Core Exercises for Seniors is an invaluable resource for anyone looking to stay fit and healthy. It provides valuable insight into the importance of core exercises, how to safely and effectively perform them, and the many benefits they can bring to seniors. The wide range of exercises and activities included in this book, along with the step-by-step instructions, make it easy to get started with core exercises. By taking the time to understand and practice core exercises for seniors, you can ensure that you have the strength, balance, and stability needed to stay active and healthy for years to come.